WALL PILATES

For

Beginners

Easy To Follow Step By Step Workout Exercise

Alessio Rossi

BOOKS BY THE SAME AUTHOR

TABLE OF CONTENTS

INTRODUCTION

WORLD OF WALL PILATES.

Jake was having trouble staying in shape. He worked at a desk job that required him to sit for long periods of time, and he was constantly tired and out of shape. Jake knew he needed to make a difference in his life, but he had no idea where to start.

While looking for fitness tips on the internet, Jake stumbled upon a book named "Wall Pilates for Beginners." Curiosity got the better of him, and he decided to click on the link to discover more. As he read the description and reviews, he became interested by the notion of Wall Pilates and how it may help him improve his fitness.

Jake ordered the book without hesitation and anticipated its arrival. When it arrived, he ripped into its pages right away.

The book is easy to read, with comprehensive explanations and step-by-step instructions. It introduced him to the world of Wall Pilates, describing the essential ideas, advantages, and how it could be tailored to novices like him.

Jake was energized and driven by what he read. He decided to build up a little workshop in his living room, knocked down a wall, and purchased a few basic tools. Using the book as a guide, he began practicing Wall Pilates moves.

It was challenging at first, but he persevered by following the beginner's routines and focusing on his breathing, alignment, and posture.

As the weeks turned into months, Jake began to detect substantial changes in his physique. His core was stronger, he was more flexible, and he felt more in control. But it wasn't only the physical advantages; his Wall Pilates practice also gave him a sense of calm and awareness.

Jake's commitment to his fitness program grew with time. He progressed from starter routines to more complex movements, all while consulting his go-to "Wall Pilates for Beginners" book. He even began personalizing his workouts to target certain regions for development.

Jake not only reached his fitness objectives, but he also acquired a passion for Wall Pilates as a result of his devotion and the recommendations in the book. He was happier, healthier, and more active than he had been in a long time. The book had proven that sometimes all it takes to make a significant change is the right information and the determination to act.

WHAT EXACTLY IS WALL PILATES?

Wall Pilates is a distinct and effective training program that combines fundamental Pilates ideas with the use of a wall for support. It is designed to help you build a strong, flexible, and balanced body while emphasizing the mind-body connection. By using the wall as a tool, you'll discover a new method to achieve your fitness goals and improve your overall well-being.

THE ADVANTAGES OF WALL PILATES

Wall Pilates provides various benefits, including core muscle strengthening, increased flexibility, and improved posture. It's a low-impact workout that can be tailored to people of various fitness levels and ages. By practicing Wall Pilates, you may enhance your physical health, mental clarity, and develop a sense of relaxation and awareness.

WHO WILL BENEFIT FROM IT?

The beauty of Wall Pilates is that it is accessible to nearly everyone. Wall Pilates may be tailored to your specific needs, whether you are a total beginner or an experienced fitness enthusiast. It's ideal for anybody looking to enhance their physical fitness, recover from injuries, decrease stress, or simply have fun while exercising.

Everyone, no matter where they are in their fitness journey, may benefit from Wall Pilates. So, let us begin this fantastic and health-improving adventure!

CHAPTER 1

UNDERSTANDING THE FUNDAMENTALS

Before we get into Wall Pilates exercises, it's vital to grasp some basic concepts. These fundamentals will form the cornerstone of your practice.

PILATES'S FUNDAMENTAL IDEA

Pilates is a practice that must follow certain regulations in order to be effective. These are the guiding principles:

1. MANAGE: Pilates emphasizes coordinated actions to engage your muscles effectively. It is not about making quick or rapid movements, but about maintaining control during each exercise. To get the most out of each exercise, concentrate on the movement and muscle engagement.

2. **ALIGNMENT:** The core of your body, also known as your "powerhouse," is the focus of Pilates. You'll learn how to get involved and strengthen this area.

3. **PRECISION:** Precision movements are more efficient. Pilates encourages exact positioning and alignment in order to activate the proper muscles while minimizing strain.

4. **FLOW:** Pilates exercises flow one after the other. The smooth, continuous motions of this method set it apart.

5. **BREATHING:** Proper breathing is vital in Pilates. It boosts your energy, oxygenates your muscles, and promotes relaxation.

REQUIRED EQUIPMENT

The fact that no extra equipment is necessarily makes Wall Pilates ideal for beginners. In truth, you just need a few simple materials to get started

1. **A WALL:** As the name indicates, you will need a wall for support and stability during your activities.

2. **COMFORTABLE CLOTHES:** Wear clothes that allows you to move freely. You don't need specific Pilates attire; simply wear something comfortable.

3. **YOGA MAT (OPTIONAL):** While not required, a yoga mat can provide additional padding for your comfort.

4. **SOCKS:** If you're training on a smooth floor, non-slip socks might be useful.

5. **KEEP AN OPEN MIND:** This isn't a tangible object, but it's vital. As you begin your Wall Pilates adventure, have an open mind and be kind with yourself.

SAFETY PRECAUTIONS

In every training routine, safety should always come first, and Wall Pilates is no exception.

1. **CONSULT A DOCTOR:** Before beginning any new exercise routine, consult with your healthcare professional if you have any medical ailments or concerns.

2. **LISTEN TO YOUR BODY**: During workouts, pay attention to how your body feels. Stop and change your position or technique if you feel pain or discomfort.

3. **START SLOWLY**: Do not jump right into advanced exercises. Begin with the fundamentals and work your way up as you gain familiarity and confidence.

4. **PROPER TECHNIQUE**: Maintain good form and technique. This makes best use of the advantages while simultaneously lowering the danger of damage.

5. **STAY HYDRATED**: To stay hydrated, drink lots of water before, during, and after your Wall Pilates exercise.

Understanding these basics is all about laying a foundation on which to build as you move through your fitness journey. So, let's get this party started!

CHAPTER 2

BREATHING AND ALIGNMENT

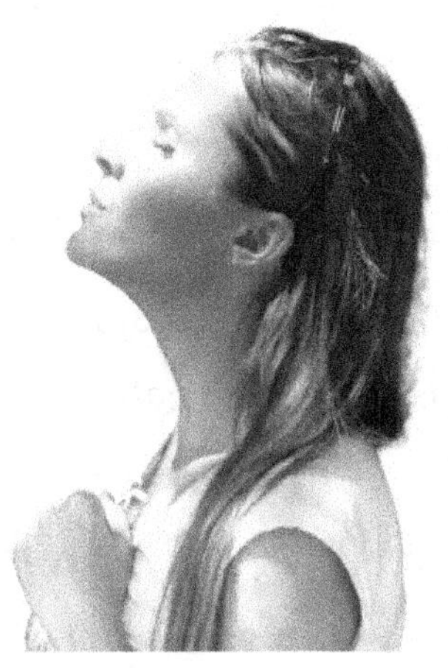

PROPER BREATHING

Wall Pilates' secret sauce is proper breathing. It's essential for integrating your mind and body and doing activities with precision and control. What you need to know about appropriate breathing in Wall Pilates is as follows:

1. **DIAPHRAGMATIC BREATHING**: Wall Pilates promotes diaphragmatic breathing, or breathing deeply into your diaphragm rather than shallowly into your chest. It improves the flow of oxygen to your muscles and keeps you centered and quiet during your practice.

2. **EXHALATION AND INHALATION**: You'll learn the proper time for breathing and exhaling throughout various exercises. This controlled breathing assists you in engaging your core muscles and achieving stability.

3. **BREATH AWARENESS**: Being aware of your breath is a key component of Wall Pilates. It's not just about breathing for the sake of breathing; it's about using your breath to improve your movement and focus your mind.

GETTING YOUR BODY IN ORDER

Alignment is the map that ensures you arrive at your fitness destination safely and successfully. This section will look at the following topics:

1. **SPINE ALIGNMENT:** Discover how to keep your spine in a neutral and healthy position when exercising. Avoiding strain and damage requires proper spine alignment.

2. **PELVIC ALIGNMENT:** Learn how to place your pelvic to support your core and keep your balance throughout motions. It's an important part of Wall Pilates.

3. **SHOULDERS AND HIPS ALIGNMENT:** Your shoulders and hips play an important role in maintaining balance and preventing muscular imbalances. You'll learn how to properly align them.

4. **MIND-BODY CONNECTION:** Alignment is about linking your mental attention with your movements as well as your physical body. You'll discover how to employ alignment to increase your focus and coordination.

Breathing efficiently and correctly align your body throughout your Wall Pilates practice. These two factors are the foundations of your road to greater strength, flexibility, and overall well-being.

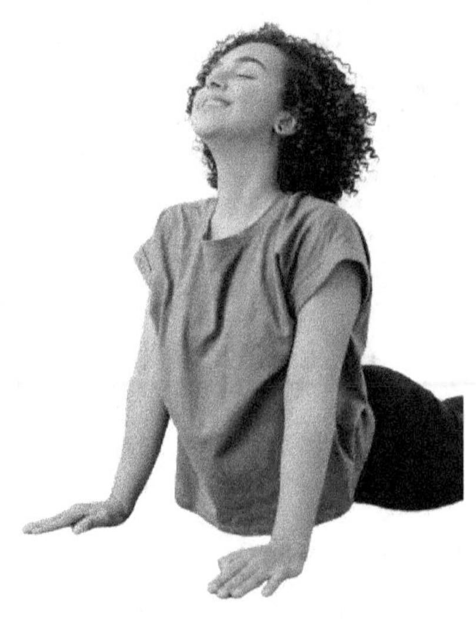

CHAPTER 3

WARM-UP AND STRETCHING

Warming up your body is important before starting any workout, even Wall Pilates. It prepares them, boosts blood flow, and minimizes the danger of damage. It also prepares you mentally for your practice.

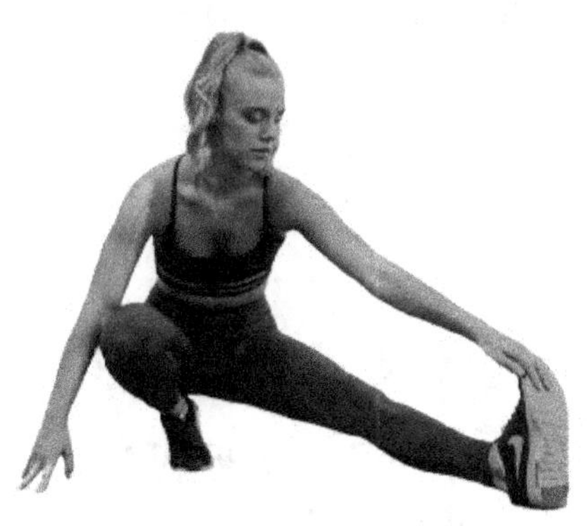

THE WARM-UP PROCEDURE

A typical Wall Pilates warm-up may include routines that slowly raise your heart rate and engage main muscle groups. The following are some fundamental warm-up exercises:

1. **MARCH IN PLACE**: Begin by marching in place with your knees lifted and your arms swinging. This raises your heart rate and prepares your muscles for action.

2. **ARM CIRCLES**: Stand with your feet hip-width apart and your arms at your sides.

Make little circles with your arms, increasing their size gradually. This helps to warm up your shoulder joints.

3. **TORSO TWISTS**: Stand with your feet hip-width apart and twist your upper body from side to side gently. This exercise warms up your spine and core.

4. **LEG SWINGS**: Find a firm support (such as a wall!) and swing one leg forward and backward gently. This gets your leg muscles and hip joints heated.

STRETCHING FOR FLEXIBILITY

Stretching improves flexibility, which is necessary for Wall Pilates. It enables you to do activities with a wider range of motion and lowers your risk of muscle strain.

1. **NECK STRETCH**: Gently tilt your head to one side for a few seconds and hold. Then, repeat on the opposite side. This stretch relaxes the muscles in your neck.

2. **SHOULDER STRETCH**: Extend one arm across your chest and pull lightly with the other hand. To extend both shoulders, switch sides.

3. **CAT-COW STRETCH**: Get down on all fours. Arch your back like a cat, then let it drop like a cow. This is excellent for extending the spine.

4. **HAMSTRING STRETCH:** Sit on the floor, one leg extended, the other bent. Keep your back straight and reach toward your toes.

5. **QUADRICEPS STRETCH:** Stand on one leg and bring your other heel toward your buttocks gently. This stretch focuses on your quads.

6. **CALF STRETCH:** Stand facing a wall, place your hands against it, and take a step back with one leg. Maintain a straight back leg while bending the front knee to stretch your calf.

You'll have a firm grasp on the warm-up and stretching exercises required for your Wall Pilates practice by the conclusion of this chapter. These principles will not only assist you in avoiding injuries, but will also increase your flexibility, laying the groundwork for a successful road to fitness and well-being.

CHAPTER 5

WALL PILATES EXERCISES FOR CORE STRENGTH

We'll look at several fundamental Wall Pilates exercises for improving core strength. The cornerstone of your body's stability and balance is a strong core. You'll be shown how to do these workouts step by step.

EXERCISE 1

WALL ROLL DOWN

STEP 1: STARTING POSITION

- Start by standing with your back to the wall.
- Maintain a hip-width distance between your feet, with your heels, hips, and shoulders contacting the wall.
- Be sure that your chin is parallel to the ground.

STEP 2: THE MOTION

1. Inhale deeply and bond your belly muscles.
2. Begin slowly sliding down the wall, one vertebra at a time, while keeping your heels, hips, and shoulders against it.
3. Exhale while rolling down, tucking your chin toward your chest.
4. Roll down as far as your flexibility will allow, ideally until your fingers contact the floor.
5. Stay in this posture for a few seconds to feel the stretch in your spine.
6. Exhale once again and begin rolling back up, reversing the process.
7. Exhale as you return to your starting posture, heels, hips, and shoulders pressed against the wall.

EXERCISE 2

WALL PLANK

STEP 1: STARTING POSITION

- Face an arm's length away from the wall.
- Place your hands on the wall, shoulder-width apart and shoulder-height.
- Take a few steps back to make an angle with your body, maintaining your feet hip-width apart.

STEP 2: THE MOTION

1. Inhale deeply and contract your abdominal muscles.
2. Exhale and push through your hands while maintaining your body straight.
3. From your head to your heels, your body should create a diagonal line.
4. Maintain this posture for as long as possible while breathing steadily.
5. Finally, exhale and take a step back, returning your body to an upright position.

EXERCISE 3

WALL LEG LIFTS

STEP 1: STARTING POSITION

- Stand approximately an arm's length away from the wall.
- Place your hands on the wall, little wider than shoulder width apart, for support.
- Maintain your balance.

STEP 2: THE MOTION

1. Inhale deeply and bond your abdominal muscles.
2. Exhale and lift one leg as high as your flexibility will allow while maintaining it straight.
3. Hold for a second, experiencing the core engagement and the extended leg.
4. Exhale and return the leg to the start position.
5. Exhale, then repeat with the opposite leg.

For greater results, remember to concentrate on your breath and technique during each exercise.

CHAPTER 5

FOCUS ON FLEXIBILITY

We will concentrate on key Wall Pilates exercises that improve flexibility. Flexibility is an important aspect of Wall Pilates because it allows you to attain a larger range of motion and prevents muscular stiffness. Let's go over these exercises one by one.

EXERCISE 1

WALL EXTEND

STEP 1: STARTING POSITION

- Stand approximately an arm's length away from the wall.
- Place your hands on the wall, shoulder-width apart and shoulder-height.

1. Inhale deeply and bond your abdominal muscles.
2. Exhale and place your hands on the wall, moving back and bending forward at the same time.
3. Keep your back straight from your heels to your hips and shoulders.
4. Notice how your spine, shoulders, and the back of your legs stretch.
5. Stay in this posture for a few minutes, focusing on deep breaths to increase the stretch.
6. Exhale softly and return to your starting posture.

EXERCISE 2

WALL LEG SWING

STEP 1: STARTING POSITION

- Stand approximately an arm's length away from the wall. Place your hands on the wall, little wider than shoulder width apart, for support. Maintain your footing.

- Inhale deeply and bond your abdominal muscles.
- Exhale and swing one leg back and forth like a swing.
- Keep your leg straight but not locked, and swing it freely.
- Swing your leg a few times, experiencing the slight stretch in your hamstrings and hip flexors.
- With each leg swing, inhale and exhale.
- Repeat the action with the opposite leg.

EXERCISE 3

WALL SPINAL TWIST

STEP 1: STARTING POSITION

- Stand approximately an arm's length away from the wall.
- Place your hands on the wall, shoulder-width apart and shoulder-height.

- Inhale deeply and bond your abdominal muscles.
- Exhale and take one step back, moving your body away from the wall.
- Keep your hands on the wall and twist your torso as much as your flexibility permits.
- Hold this posture for a few breaths, allowing your spine and chest to extend.
- Exhale and inhale to increase the stretch.
- Return to the beginning posture and twist on the opposite side.

These Wall Pilates flexibility exercises are intended to increase your range of motion, reduce muscular tension, and improve your general mobility. Include them in your program on a regular basis to get the full advantages of Wall Pilates and a more flexible and functioning body. Remember to take deep breaths and complete these exercises with control and focus.

CHAPTER 5

FOCUS ON BALANCE

Balance is essential for overall well-being, stability, and coordination. Let's go over these exercises one by one.

EXERCISE 1

WALL SQUAT

STEP 1: STARTING POSITION

- Place your back to the wall and your feet hip-width apart.
- Your heels, hips, and shoulders should all be in contact with the wall.
- Maintain your hands on your hips.

STEP 2: THE MOTION

- Take a deep breath in and engage your core.
- Exhale and bend your knees to lower your body into a squat position. Assume you're seated in an invisible chair.

- Keep your knees from going beyond your toes and your heels, hips, and shoulders against the wall.

- Hold the squat for a few breaths, feeling the thighs and core engage.

- Hold the squat while inhaling and exhaling.

- Return to the start posture by pushing through your heels.

EXERCISE 2

WALL LUNGE

STEP 1: STARTING POSITION

- Face the wall and place your hands shoulder-width apart on it for support.

- Take a couple steps back, keeping your feet hip-width apart.

STEP 2: THE MOTION

- Take a deep breath in and engage your core.

- Exhale, then lower into a lunge by bending your front leg and lowering your hips toward the ground.

- Make sure your back leg is straight behind you.

- Maintain balance on the ball of your back foot while keeping your front knee in line with your ankle.

- Hold the lunge for a few breaths, noticing how your leg muscles extend and activate.

- Hold the lunge while inhaling and exhaling.

- Return to the start posture by pushing through your front heel, then swap legs and repeat.

EXERCISE 3

WALL BRIDGE

STEP 1: STARTING POSITION

- Lie on your back, knees bent, and feet hip-width apart.

- Place your arms at your sides, palms facing down.

- Your heels, hips, and shoulders should all be in contact with the wall.

STEP 2: THE MOTION

- Take a deep breath in and engage your core.
- Exhale, then lift your hips off the ground in a straight line from your shoulders to your knees.
- Maintain the bridge posture by squeezing your glutes and engaging your core.
- Hold the bridge for a few breaths, feeling the glutes and core engage.
- Breathe in and out while holding the bridge.
- Return to the start posture by lowering your hips to the ground.

These Wall Pilates balancing exercises are intended to enhance your stability and coordination. Including these exercises into your regimen on a regular basis can help you establish a strong sense of balance and improve your general body control. Remember to breathe deeply, keep perfect form, and complete these exercises with control and attention.

CHAPTER 4

FULL-BODY WALL PILATES WORKOUTS

Wall Pilates routines for all fitness levels, including beginners, intermediate, and advanced. We'll go over each routine one by one.

BEGINNERS ROUTINE

FIRST STEP: WARM-UP

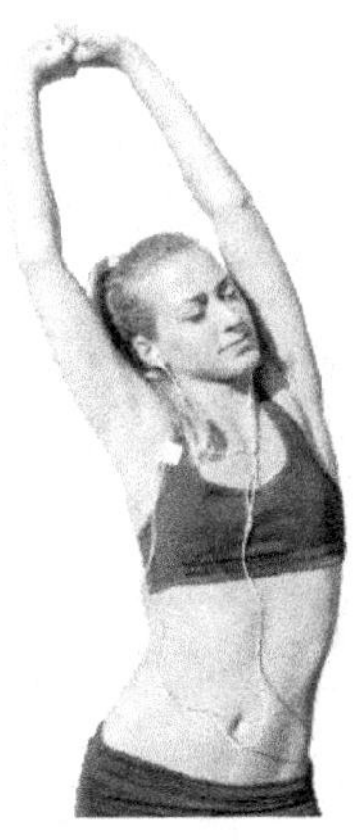

- Start by completing simple warm-up exercises like as walking in place.
- rotating your arms in circles, and slowly twisting your upper body.
- Spend 5-7 minutes preparing your body for the workout.

STEP 2: WALL ROLL DOWN

1. Place your back against the wall.
2. Breathe in deeply and grip your stomach.
3. Breathe out as you bend down towards the floor, then inhale as you rise back up.

STEP 3: WALL SQUAT

1. Perform the wall squat that we discussed in the balance part.
2. Hold the squat for 30 seconds to 1 minute, focusing on technique and breathing.

STEP 4: LEG LIFTS ON THE WALL

1. Place your hands on the wall for support.
2. Straighten one leg in front of you, then lower it.
3. Repeat 10-12 times on each leg.

STEP 5: RELAX

- Stretch gently toward the end.
- Stretch the muscles you worked on during the program for 15-30 seconds at a time.

INTERMEDIATE ROUTINE

FIRST STEP: WARM-UP

- warm up with more energetic activities like jumping jacks, lifting your knees up high, and lunges.
- Warm up for around 7-10 minutes.

STEP 2: WALL PLANK

- Stand in a plank stance facing the wall.
- Maintain this position for 30 seconds to 1 minute while maintaining your body straight.

STEP 3: WALL LUNGE

- Perform the wall lunges as described before.
- Perform 12-15 lunges on each leg.

STEP 4: WALL BRIDGE

- Perform the wall bridge exercise while lying on your back.
- Keep the bridge in place for 30 seconds to 1 minute.

STEP 5: RELAX

- Finish with gradual stretches for all of your major muscles.
- holding each for 20-45 seconds

ADVANCE ROUTINE

STEP 1: WARM-UP

Warm-up with more difficult activities like hard jumping jacks, mountain climbers, and dynamic stretches. Warm up for around 10-15 minutes.

STEP 2: CHANGES FROM WALL ROLL DOWN TO WALL PLANK

- Start by rolling down the wall.
- Transition into a smooth wall plank and hold for 15-30 seconds.

- Return to the down position on the wall.

STEP 3: ADVANCED WALL PILATES EXERCISES

Combine more difficult workouts such as advanced wall squats, dynamic leg swings, and twisting planks.

STEP 4: LEG LIFTS ON THE WALL

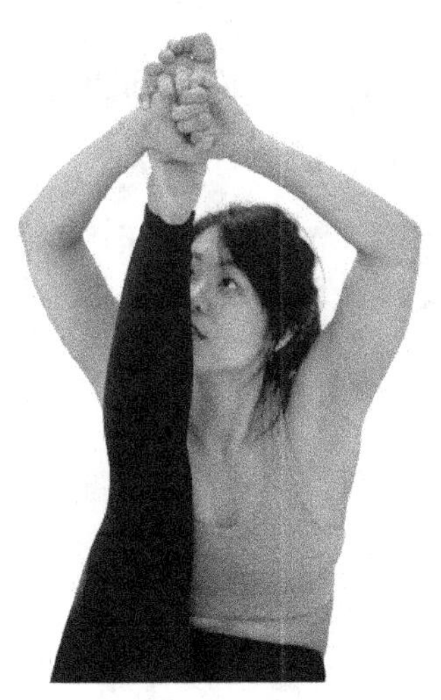

To make wall leg lifts more difficult, use resistance bands. Perform 15-20 repetitions on each leg.

STEP 5: RELAX.

- Finish with a thorough stretch, holding it for 30-60 seconds.
- Stretch all of the muscles that you worked during the workout.

These full-body Wall Pilates exercises are designed for people of all fitness levels. Depending on how you feel, adjust the duration and amount of reps. To ensure a safe and successful workout, always perform each motion with proper form and control.

CHAPTER 5

ADAPTING WALL PILATES TO YOUR SPECIFIC NEEDS

We'll discuss how to modify Wall Pilates to meet a variety of demands, including those of elders, persons recuperating from injuries, and those seeking stress reduction. Let's take a look at each adaption one by one.

SENIOR WALL PILATES

STEP 1: LIGHT WARM-UP

- Start by gradually warming up.
- Slowly move and engage in exercises such as sitting and elevating your legs or creating gentle circles with your arms.
- To aid with balance, lean against the wall during workouts.
- Modify your actions so that they do not put too much strain on your joints.

- To help you relax, focus on breathing deeply and gently.

STEP 2: SEATED WALL WORKOUTS

- Sit comfortably and raise one knee at a time as if marching against a wall.
- Sit down and gently press your hands on the wall to train your upper body.

STEP 3: RELAX.

Finish with easy stretches while sitting, ensuring that you are comfortable and calm.

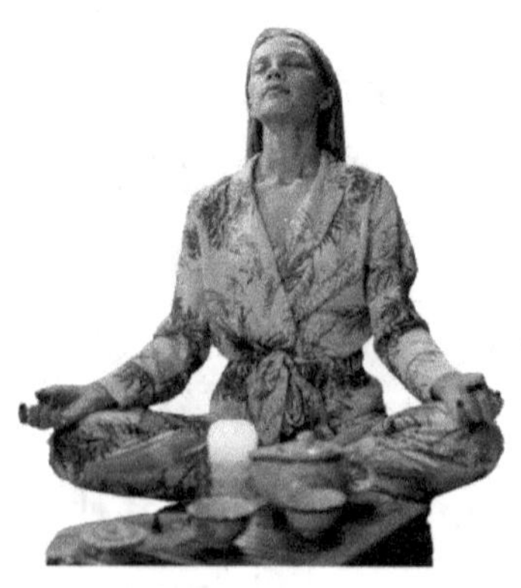

INJURY THERAPY WITH WALL PILATES

STEP 1: CONSULT A PROFESSIONAL

Before you start, consult with a doctor or physical therapist to determine any limitations or alterations that may be required for your rehabilitation.

STEP 2: GO SLOWLY

- Start with light warm-up exercises to get your blood circulating.
- Select the appropriate wall Pilates routines that will not aggravate your ailment. if necessary, replace them.
- concentrate on doing it right by making sure that you are performing each action correctly.
- start slowly and progress to tougher workouts as you gain strength.
- Finish with stretches for the improved region and a gradual cool-down to allow your body recuperate.

STRESS RELIEVING WALL PILATES

- Start with a warm-up that allows you to focus on the present moment.

- Make soft movements and take deep breaths.

- Spend some time practicing gentle breathing techniques.

- Perform gentle stretches, giving special attention to areas of tension.

- Perform a wall plank while focusing on your body. Consider each muscle you're utilizing.

- To help you relax, try sitting wall stretches.

- Finish with some relaxing stretches to make you feel more at ease and less anxious.

By adapting Wall Pilates to specific requirements, more individuals may benefit from it. We ensure that everyone may benefit by adapting the technique for elders, persons in rehab, and those seeking stress alleviation. Always pay attention to your body and make adjustments as needed.

CHAPTER 6

MAINTAINING CONSISTENCY AND PROGRESS

Let's talk about how to stick with your Wall Pilates program and keep pushing forward in this chapter. We'll divide it into three steps.

1. SETTING OBJECTIVES

STEP 1: DETERMINE YOUR GOALS

- Consider your goals for Wall Pilates, whether they are to get stronger, more flexible, or simply to feel better.
- Make your objectives clear and explicit. For example, you may try to hold a wall board for a set period of time.

STEP 2: TAKE DOWN

- Goals that lead to your long-term ambitions. These are things that you can accomplish in the short term.

- Make sure your objectives are practical and appropriate for your fitness level and time commitment.

STEP 3: MAINTAIN YOUR MOTIVATION

- Visualize yourself achieving your objectives. This might assist you in remaining motivated.
- Commemorate the small victories along the road. It keeps you motivated to take the next step.

2.MONITORING PROGRESS

STEP 1: MAINTAIN A JOURNAL

- Take notes on the exercises you completed, how long you did them for, and anything else you observed.
- Keep track of when you accomplish anything, such as holding a position for a longer period of time or doing a more difficult activity.

STEP 2: CONSISTENT CHECK UP

- Monitor your progress on a regular basis, perhaps every few weeks. Check in on how you're doing.
- As your fitness level improves, you may need to adjust your goals. As you go, make adjustments.

STEP 3: PAY ATTENTION TO YOUR BODY

- Recognize what your body is telling you. Change or skip workouts if anything doesn't seem right.
- Progress isn't simply about statistics. Celebrate feeling better, having better posture, or simply having fun with your workouts.

1. MODIFYING YOUR ROUTINE

STEP 1: VALIDATE CONSISTENCY

- Determine how frequently you exercise. Are you following through on your plans?
- Check to see whether there are moments when sticking to your schedule is simpler or more difficult.

STEP 2: CHANGES MUST BE ACCEPTED

- Accept that life changes. Change your schedule to reflect what's going on in your life.
- Your schedule may need to modify depending on factors such as how much energy you have or how stressed you are.

STEP 3: CONTINUE FORWARD

- As you become more accustomed to your routine, gradually increase the difficulty. Experiment with increasingly difficult exercises.
- Keep things fresh by experimenting with new variations of activities. It keeps your body on edge.

Setting specific objectives, tracking your progress, and changing your program as required ensures that your Wall Pilates practice remains pleasurable and beneficial. Consistency and adaptability will enable you to continue improving and feeling good.

CHAPTER 7

HEALTHY LIFESTYLE SUGGESTIONS

We'll look at helpful hints for living a healthy lifestyle, such as diet, sleep, recuperation, and mixing Wall Pilates with other activities. Let's take each aspect one at a time.

DIET AND NUTRITION

STEP 1: EAT A WELL-BALANCED DIET

- Eat a range of fruits, vegetables, complete grains, and lean meats.
- Maintain a balanced nutritional intake by paying attention to portion sizes.

STEP 2: HYDRATION

- Drink water throughout the day to stay hydrated.
- For improved overall health, limit your intake of sugary beverages.

STEP 3: PRE-EXERCISE NUTRITION

- Eat a nutritious lunch or snack 1-2 hours before your Wall Pilates practice.
- Carbohydrates should be prioritized for energy, while protein should be included for muscular support.

SLEEP AND RECUPERATION

STEP 1: MAKE SLEEP A PRIORITY

- Maintain a consistent sleep pattern for greater quality sleep.
- Make your sleeping area comfy and relaxing.

STEP 2: POST-EXERCISE RECOVERY

- After your Wall Pilates workout, give your body a quick rest.
- Rehydrate post-workout for maximum recovery.

- Take rest days as needed to enable your body to recuperate.
- On rest days, consider mild exercises like walking or easy stretching.

COLLABORATION WITH OTHER ACTIVITIES

STEP 1: THE ADVANTAGES OF CROSS-TRAINING

- For total fitness, combine Wall Pilates with other exercises such as walking, cycling, or swimming.
- Break up your routine with new workouts to avoid boredom.

STEP 2: LOOK FOR FUN ACTIVITIES

- Participate in activities that you like, supporting a holistic approach to well-being.
- Participate in group courses or work out with friends to make exercise more fun.

- Create a regular training routine that allows for a variety of activities.
- Be aware of your body's signals and alter your activity accordingly.

By adopting these suggestions into your daily routine, you will improve the overall efficacy of your Wall Pilates practice and contribute to your general well-being. Balancing diet, prioritizing sleep, and varied activities lay the groundwork for a healthy, long-term lifestyle.

CHAPTER 8

SOLUTIONS TO COMMON CHALLENGES

We'll look at practical answers to typical problems that may arise during your Wall Pilates journey. We'll talk about overcoming Obstacles, discomfort, and staying motivated.

OVERCOMING OBSTACLES

STEP 1: ASSESS YOUR ROUTINE

- Pay close attention to what you're doing throughout your Wall Pilates workouts. Do you have any workouts that you've been performing for a while?

- Make sure your workouts are demanding enough. Your body might become used to the same degree of hardship.

STEP 2: INTRODUCE VARIETIES

- Introduce some new Wall Pilates routines to work on various muscles.
- Gradually increase the difficulty of your workout.

STEP 3: ESTABLISH PROGRESSIVE GOALS

- Adjust your fitness objectives as you go.
- Recognize and celebrate tiny victories to keep oneself motivated.

SORENESS MANAGEMENT

STEP 1: RECOGNIZE NORMAL DISCOMFORT

- It's natural to be sore after working out.
- Know the difference between normal soreness and acute or long-lasting pain.

STEP 2: PRIORITIZE RECOVERY STRATEGIES

- On days when you don't perform Pilates, try mild exercises like walking or easy stretching.
- Include diet high in protein and anti-inflammatory characteristics.

STEP 3: GRADUAL INCREASE

- Gradually increase the intensity of your wall Pilates movements to allow your muscles to adjust.
- If you're regularly hurting, try slowing down and focusing on executing exercises with proper technique.

MAINTAINING MOTIVATION

STEP 1: REVIEW YOUR OBJECTIVES

- Consider why you began Wall Pilates and what you hope to achieve.
- Imagine the benefits of sticking to your exercise goals.

STEP 2: VARY YOUR ROUTINE

- With different Wall Pilates routines to keep things fresh.
- Try out new routines or activities to keep oneself interested and minimize monotony.

STEP 3: ACCOUNTABILITY AND ASSISTANCE

- Team up with a friend or attend a group class to encourage one another.
- Share your accomplishments with others to foster a supportive environment.

By implementing these methods, you will be more prepared to face problems, resulting in a positive and pleasurable Wall Pilates experience. Changing your regimen, dealing with discomfort properly, and remaining motivated all contribute to a successful and long-term fitness journey.

CHAPTER 9

WHAT HAPPENS NEXT IN WALL PILATES?

We will discuss what happens after the beginner level in Wall Pilates. We'll look at advanced methods and tailored routines to help you develop your practice.

ADVANCED METHODS

STEP 1: LEARN THE FUNDAMENTALS

- Make sure you understand the fundamental Wall Pilates routines.
- Pay great attention to having proper form and performing actions with control.

STEP 2: ADVANCING IN WALL PILATES

- Begin by including more difficult types of workouts to push yourself.
- For a more fluid exercise, try flowing smoothly between different Wall Pilates postures.

STEP 3: HIGHLIGHTING THE CORE

- Include workouts that target your core muscles in both the front and back.
- Include dynamic stability exercises to increase core strength and control.

SPECIFIC WORKOUTS

STEP 1: DETERMINE YOUR OBJECTIVES

- Determine exactly what you want from your workouts, such as being more flexible, stronger, or targeting certain muscles.
- Tailor your exercises to your specific requirements and tastes.

STEP 2: SPECIFIC WALL PILATES WORKOUTS

- Design exercises that focus on increasing flexibility. Stretches and exercises that improve flexibility should be included.
- Create a plan that focuses on increasing muscular strength and power by performing difficult workouts.

STEP 3: INCLUDE OTHER TYPES OF EXERCISE

- To provide diversity, combine Wall Pilates with other workouts such as yoga or resistance training.
- Create routines that address several components of fitness, such as cardio, strength, and flexibility.

Taking Wall Pilates beyond the fundamentals entails learning advanced techniques and adapting your exercises to your unique goals. Whether it's adding complexity to your exercises, focusing on core strength, or developing customized routines, these stages can help you advance your practice and achieve your fitness goals.

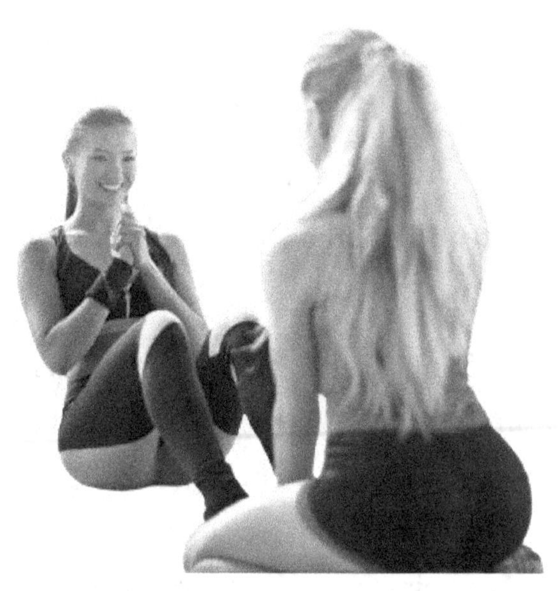

7-DAY WALL PILATES TRAINING SCHEDULE FOR BEGINNERS

DAY 1:

ESTABLISHING A FOUNDATION

1. 3 sets of 10 repetitions of wall roll down
2. Wall Plank: Hold for 20 seconds, then repeat three times more.
3. Wall Squat: three sets of twelve repetitions

DAY 2:

STRETCH AND UNWIND

1. Wall Stretch: Hold for 30 seconds, then repeat twice more.
2. Wall Leg Swing: three sets of fifteen swings each leg
3. Wall Spinal Twist: Perform two sets of 12 twists on each side.

DAY 3:

CORE STABILIZATION

1. Wall Plank: Hold for 30 seconds, then repeat three times more.
2. Wall Leg Lifts: three sets of twelve lifts per leg
3. Wall Bridge: two sets of fifteen repetitions

DAY 4:

COMPLETE BODY ENGAGEMENT

1. Wall Squat: 3 sets of 15 reps.
2. Wall Roll Down: three sets of twelve repetitions
3. Leg Lifts on the Wall: 2 sets of 10 lifts each leg.

DAY 5:

INTERMEDIATE TEST

1. Transition from wall plank to push-up: 3 sets of 8 transitions
2. Wall Lunge: three sets of ten lunges each leg.
3. Wall Spinal Twist with Leg Extension: Perform two sets of 12 twists on each side.

DAY 6:

STRESS ON FLEXIBILITY

1. Wall Stretch: Hold for 40 seconds, then repeat twice more.
2. Wall Leg Swing: three sets of twenty swings each leg
3. Wall Roll Down with Forward Bend: two sets of ten repetitions each.

DAY 7:

MINDFUL MOVEMENT

1. Rotating Wall Plank: 3 sets of 12 rotations
2. Calf Raise with Wall Squat: 3 sets of 15 repetitions
3. Wall Pilates Flow: Perform a continuous series of Wall Roll Down, Wall Plank, and Wall Leg Lifts.

Remember to listen to your body, alter exercises as required, and have fun learning about the advantages of Wall Pilates. Please contact our support staff if you have any complaints or queries. Good luck with your Pilates!

CONCLUSION

As you complete "Wall Pilates for Beginners," we'd want to convey our appreciation for joining us on this fitness adventure.

Your dedication to studying and practicing Wall Pilates is admirable, and we hope you found this tutorial useful.

We request you to leave a review and share your ideas. Your opinion not only helps us grow, but it also helps other fitness enthusiasts make educated decisions regarding their own fitness path.

If you have any issues or want additional assistance, please contact our support staff via email Rossihelpdesk@gmail.com.

We're here to help and answer any questions you may have.

Thank you for taking the time to read "Wall Pilates for Beginners."

We hope that this resource has helped you understand and enjoy Wall Pilates, promoting a better and more active lifestyle.

Best wishes for continuing success and joy on your fitness journey!

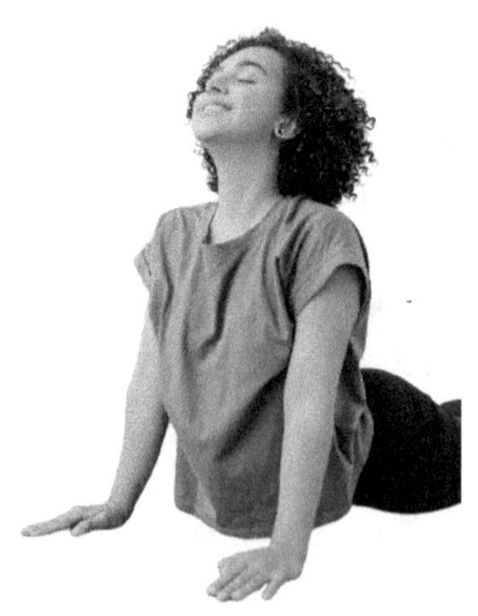